THE REGISTERED NURSE

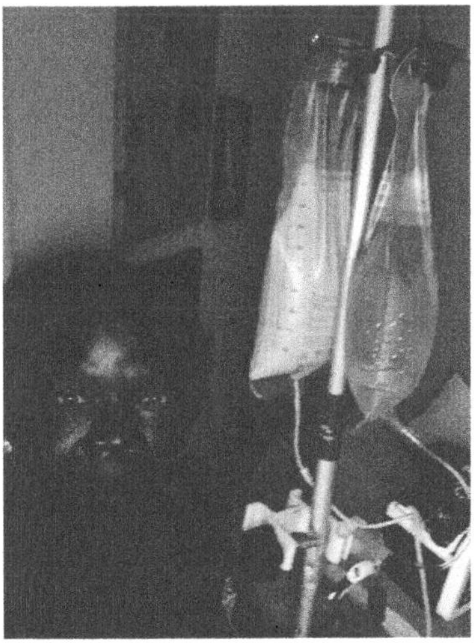

Anne Dada

Anne Dada

First Edition

Published by The Lighthouse books, Agape Inc.

For information regarding permission, write to:

The Lighthouse,15600 E. Caley Pl, Centennial,

CO 80016.

ISBN: 978-1-950320-05-9

Visit us at:

www.thelighthousebooks.com

Printed in the USA

Anne Dada

FOREWORD

Two little girls were in their front yard playing, clapping and jumping, happy in the eventide, oblivious to the world and the danger lurking in the very grounds on which they played. Suddenly, one of the girls screamed and fell to the ground holding on to her foot with blood everywhere. The other sister ran into the house to fetch their mother who came out to see what had happened, and upon seeing the blood, the mother ran back in to get a first aid kit to clean the wound and stop the bleeding. The injured girl had stepped on several nails left behind by workers that had done some repair work on the house a few days earlier. She was taken to the hospital where she had two experiences that would stay with her for life and helped to shape her future career.

The wounded girl had never visited such big buildings before; she was intimidated by the sheer size of the hospital. She clung to the arms of her mother crying. In the emergency room the look on her face reflected the terror she felt inside.

Two strangers entered the exam room: the doctor dressed in white from head to toe and a nurse in scrubs. Seeing that this little girl was crying and scared, the nurse, (the girl would describe her later as an angel sent to take care of her), spoke kindly to her and gave her some candies. The nurse took her from her mother until she became calm and quiet again. After she was seen by the doctor, the nurse administered the prescribed medications.

The nurse expertly administered an injection that the little girl only whimpered once before it was over. By the time all her treatments were completed, she was sound asleep in her mother's arms, waking shortly after they arrived home.

As the little girl grew older, she knew exactly what she what she wanted to do for a life career. Her recurring flash backs to her experience at the hospital many years before profoundly impacted her decision to become a nurse. She told her mother that she wanted to be like the "angel" that took care of her.

The story of the registered nurse often does not start at admission into college or nursing school. Like this young girl, many begin to have dreams of becoming a nurse from younger years either from the experiences they had or found themselves thrust into it. These influential life experiences help them develop their passion for the profession of nursing.

Whatever informs the individual's decision to go into nursing, no amount of preparation through college or nursing school meets the reality of nursing practice in real times. This book therefore attempts to paint a brief picture of the life of a registered nurse at work in real time. It hopefully gives the "nurse-dreamer" a glimpse into the real world of nursing. This, together with years of schooling, should help equip the individual for a life in nursing practice as a caring, passionate and professional nurse. The experiences shared in this book applies more specifically to surgical medical nursing in an acute care setting.

Happy reading.

DEDICATION

This book is dedicated first to God Almighty for His unwavering love for me, for the gift of life, and grace to write this book, and to my senior Pastor-Bishop Israel Ade Ajala of Kingdom Connection Christian Center, Aurora Colorado, for his heart to see his members succeed, therefore his never ending push and encouragement to all, to aim and leap high. To my parents whose love, passion, and effort, to educate their children has been inspiring. Lastly to my dear children and husband for their care and support. I love you all

CONTENTS

CHAPTER ONE:

The New Nurse Graduate

Three to four years of education in a college or nursing school prepares you for your board examination and practice as a Registered Nurse. Once you pass the examination, you become registered in your state of intended practice. Then finally the job search starts. This may take series of job interviews and offers before you make your choice of where to practice.

Once the start date is set, you go in for an orientation. As a new nurse graduate, many facilities have the new nurse graduate program that usually includes the mission and vision of the facility. This tells you about the culture of practice at that facility with the expectation that you would follow similar practice.

Of course, you would have decided at your interview what shift you want to work when you start, or what kind of shifts they offer at the facility and that which best suits you.

There are varieties of shifts in clinical care usually twelve-hour shifts as follows: Day shift from 7am to 7:30pm with a

30minuites break, or the night shift from 7pm to 7:30am also with a 30minutes break, and depending on the unit, other hours may apply.

You could do only one or the other and in some facilities, you rotate from one to the other. How shifts are run is dependent on each facility. With twelve-hour shifts, you are mandated to work three days a week.

Following orientation, the new nurse graduate program starts. This is where you learn the synopsis of clinical nursing practice in general, from day to day and from one scenario to another, using critical thinking skills. At this stage, there is no interaction with patients, but there are simulations with manikins that are programmed to behave like humans in real life situations. This program usually lasts six weeks, again, the duration is facility specific. After successfully completing the training you are then ready to join the work force. This is when the RN's career starts.

The Nursing career has very vast areas of discipline ranging from: acute care that deals with medical surgical patients primarily, to orthopedics, pediatrics, labor and delivery, intensive care, the operating room (OR) and psychiatry among others.

The experience gained in acute care setting after about one to two years of practice is usually sufficient to help the individual decide the area of specific nursing discipline he/she may want to pursue long-term. This book is recommended for beginners in nursing practice.

CHAPTER TWO

Preceptorship

Welcome to the real world of nursing.

Preceptorship for new nurse graduates is usually between six to eight weeks, or twelve weeks for the operating room department in some facilities. This however may vary from facility to facility.

The preceptorship is a program where the new nurse graduate works with an experienced RN to witness and practice firsthand, nursing as an employee. The individual goes through the skills laboratory where he/she is taken through the common skills in nursing practice. For example, inserting a Foley catheter, inserting intravenous catheter, setting up feeding pumps, PCA pumps (Patient Controlled Analgesia) etc.

By the second week, he/she begins to take a patient load, starting with one patient and increasing to six by the last week of preceptorship. By the way, most facilities have a nurse-patient ratio of 1-6, depending on the department.

It is important to know here that proficiency of the preceptor and her ability to precept well will reflect on the preceptee, that is the new nurse graduate. Also, of note is the demeanor (attitude) of the new nurse graduate at the beginning of preceptorship and the development of his/her self-confidence as the weeks go by. At the end of the program, he/she should be ready to roll.

Individuals have different learning curves. If at the end of a preceptorship, the nurse in training feels unprepared to work without supervision, then they are given an extension of two or more weeks. The extension is judged accordingly. This will allow the new nurse to be provided with further training so that they will succeed as a nurse.

CHAPTER THREE

Ready to Roll

The Value of Critical thinking in nursing

For a nurse to become proficient in the care of patients and have good patient care outcomes, the critical thinking skills must be excellent and on point, as it may be life or death to the patient. Although the nurse graduate may be equipped with clinical skills in college, critical thinking is learned on the job. It improves with practice and requires that the entire world and content of nursing (including ideas, theories, and concept of nursing) is put into consideration in each patient's condition. Critical thinkers therefore need to be precise, complete, logical, accurate, clear and fair with all the activities they do: talking, documenting or actual performance of their duties (NurseJournal.org, 2019).

The Blue Book (my terminology) for nurses is the Nursing Policy and Procedure(P&P) is available in all healthcare facilities for reference when in doubt. Rather than making any error of policy or procedure, it serves the RN better to clarify from this document before going ahead with the intended care. All new nurse graduates should be thus informed during orientation or preceptorship.

A typical day in the medical-surgical unit.

0653-0700: RN clocks in to work

Picks up his/her assigned patients' SBAR to look through, and walks with the signing off RN (Registered Nurse) to the patient's rooms for report on how the previous shift went. SBAR is a tool nurses use to assess patients and develop their care plans.

SBAR is an acronym that stands for the following:

S- Situation:

What is going on with the patient right now? Here the nurse identifies himself or herself to the patient. The nurse explains in a concise manner what the problem is as received in the report.

B- Background:

What is the background on this patient? How did we get to this point? The nurse reviews the chart, anticipates questions and states the relevant medical issues.

A- Assessment:

What do you think the issue is? Why are you concerned? The nurse provides their observations and evaluation of the patient's current state, including current nursing index of vital signs and other relevant symptoms.

R- Recommendation:

What should be done to resolve the current situation? What do you recommend as measures to resolve the situation?

The SBAR is also a tool of communication with the doctors caring for patients.

The nurses introduce themselves to the patient and briefly discuss the previous shift. This includes: the present situation of the patient, the background, assessment, and recommendation. This process is to get the patient acquainted with the new RN allowing the new nurse to get involved and contribute to their own plan of care for the day. This allows the patient to have expectations of their care so they are not surprised by actions taken by the nurse.

In order for the RN to provide holistic care, the nurse is responsible to the patient as a caregiver, teacher, counsellor, advocate, and liaison person with family members and more. The RN is told what has been done and what still needs be done as a continuum of care.

After taking report, the nurse develops a plan of care for each patient assigned. The nurse reviews the patients' laboratory records, pending examinations, due medications. The nurse prioritizes his/ her plan, by order of need, the patient to see first, and what care to perform. At this time, the RN has gathered all available bio-data on each patient that includes: vital signs, intake and output, height and weight (where appropriate), tele-monitor result and so on. Then he/she goes from patient to patient to do a physical assessment on each of them noting findings and determining how to implement care as appropriate. At this time, the nurse will complete what is commonly called the 6Ps of need. The goal is to meet several or all of the 6Ps, as necessary.

The 6P's include: Putty, Pain, Possessions, Position, Pick-up, and Pumps.

Putty-

Does the patient need to use the bathroom? If so, the nurse or her assistant, the CNA, takes the patient to the bathroom or the bedside commode (BSC). The BSC is a urinal or bedpan, allowing the patient to have an easy access to the bathroom.

In incontinent patients, the RN ensures that the patient has neither soiled nor wet themselves and proceeds to change them as needed.

At this point the RN can call for help from her colleagues if she can't perform this care immediately or alone.

Pain-

Is the patient in pain?

The RN assesses the patient. The nurse uses their own judgement to determine necessary intervention for pain relief. The patient may need medications, cold or heat therapy, a drink of water or any other request that can be met within reason.

Nurses can give medication while other non-clinical care tasks are delegated to the nurse's team members.

Positioning-

Some patients require a change to their position to become more comfortable. While others may be on a turning schedule. This is common in unconscious or semi-conscious patients or those who cannot help themselves. A 2-hourly turn schedule means the patient must be repositioned on the hour.

Positioning is important because in addition to being comfortable, it prevents patients from developing pressure sores.

Pick-up-

When patients drop items on the floor, they may need help to pick them up. Even when the patient is able to pick up the object, helping the patient, prevents the risk of them falling and sustaining other injuries.

If the RN observes there are things in the room that need picked-up, the nurse can kindly offer his/her assistance. This keeps the room as clean and tidy as possible, knowing this is home for the patients as long as they are on admission.

Pumps-

Each patient's room has intravenous pumps for use to deliver fluids or medications intravenously. When pumps are in use, they are programmed to beep, alerting the RN of a malfunction. The beeping sound can be disturbing for the patient, prevent sleep, or is plainly annoying. When the RN notices the beeping pumps on rounds, the nurse will fix it. Or if discovered by the assistant, a nurse will be called to fix it.

Evidence based practice identifies that patients are more comfortable when they have all the 6ps met. The RN is responsible to ensure preemptive care of patients during hourly rounds to find out their needs before they call. This is known to decrease the frequency of call lights and fall risks in patients.

After the RN has drawn up a plan of care, he/she proceeds to implement care by giving medications and ensures that patients' intravenous accesses are clean, dry, intact and up to date. The rule of thumb is for IVs to last four days from insertion barring incidences like infiltrations, inflammation (evidenced by swelling), pain, redness etc. These need immediate attention to change the sites.

Caring continues until about noon when the RN can go for a 30-minutes lunch break. The nurse has a "buddy" to take care of his/her patients until they return and vice-versa.

Admission, discharge and end of life processes.

Of all the nursing processes to implement, perhaps the most important are the admission and discharge of patients and the end of life procedures.

On a typical day, the nurse-patient ratio is 1-5 on day shift and 1-6 at night. Every nurse should therefore be ready for at least one admission and one discharge on his/her shift.

Admission

Oftentimes, a new patient comes in from the emergency department, but other times, patient may be a direct admit from doctor offices, or even a transfer from another facility. Regardless of where the patient comes from, according to the hospital policy, the receiving nurse is informed of the admission and given report on the patient. This is to help the nurse prepare to receive the patient by getting the room ready and attend to other relevant needs. The admission process is key to the care and outcome of care of the patient.

A detailed assessment of the patient's physical, social, spiritual and psychological being may reveal other subtle symptoms that the patient may not have reported to the doctor at first contact.

The nurse will need to do a head to toe assessment that includes all the body systems from: neurological, neurovascular, cardiac, respiratory, musculoskeletal, ear, eye and throat, integumentary, gastro-intestinal, immunologic, hepatobiliary and pancreatic, renal and urinary, and endocrine and metabolic. At this point the nurse will make a diagnosis and prepare to intervene as appropriate. The nurse will document all findings and may need to inform the attending physician for any new findings.

A list of the patient's home medication is also done at this time, noting the address of the dispensing pharmacy for contact as needed. The physician reviews the medication list and orders medication that need to be continued on admission, in addition to any other orders that the nurse must implement.

Discharge

On discharge, depending on where the patient is going, maybe home or other facilities, the process is per the hospital policy. It includes getting all relevant documentation ready to send with the patient, the medication list and any prescriptions. The patient is also educated on their current situation including: concerning symptoms to report for immediate medical attention, lifestyle changes and follow-up appointments with the (PCP) Primary Care Provider or a specific specialty.

For discharges to other facilities, the medical report is called ahead to the receiving nurse. The receiving nurse is then told the expected time of arrival allowing them time to prepare to receive the patient. Transportation is arranged and a brief report on basis of need to know is given to the transporters so as not to breech patients' privacy.

End of life process

The end of life process is implemented when a patient dies. This is typically the most traumatic task for a nurse, especially if it is not anticipated.

The nurse must inform members of the family, who in most cases will come to the hospital and be told of events leading to the death of the patient. Doctors are also involved in this process. Family psychological needs are met at this time and a designated certified staff will discuss with the family if the patient is an organ donor.

Arrangements are made with a funeral home, donor alliance and death registry are called and if the patient is qualified, the coroner is informed.

Family is allowed to spend as much time as they desire with the patient to bid farewell before the body is moved out of the room to the mortuary or by the funeral home.

The same process occurs with patients on comfort care only. Comfort care is for patients whose end of life is anticipated.

Admissions and discharges can occur at any time during the shift and the nurse would determine how she can complete this process amid her care of other patients. Teamwork is necessary as it helps facilitate a smooth progress of all that needs be done in a timely manner, including situations of occurrence of death.

Doctors' orders are updated in the computer from time to time and it is the responsibility of the RN to check for orders throughout the shift for implementation. In situations where there is a change in a patient's condition for the worse, the RN calls out to the attending doctor using the SBAR to inform of the patient's situation and recommendations. When physicians give telephone orders, the RN enters such orders in the computer appropriately and goes on to implement them.

After lunch, the RN continues to do hourly rounds on patients, needs are met as needed, and care continues until the shift is over. The next shift arrives and shift report and handing over is done all over again as was done at the beginning of the shift.

In some situations, however, patients sometimes may take a sudden turn for the worse that is life threatening. It may present as impairment of circulation or respiration. This calls for a multidisciplinary approach of care at the same time in the form of a code.

CHAPTER FOUR

First Code Blue experience.

First Code Blue experience.

Facilities have some unusual situations color coded and established as policies. All members of staff are expected to know their roles in these codes.

For example, code blue informs staff that a patient is in a life-threatening situation and at risk to die. Therefore, there is immediate medical intervention to resuscitate. This code is paged overhead so that everyone can hear it and all assigned members of staff come together at patient's bedside to give necessary resuscitative care. Two outcomes are expected; either the patient is revived and is taken to a higher level of care unit, usually the intensive care unit (ICU), until the patient is stabilized, or dies.

The first code blue experience of the new nurse graduate can be emotionally traumatic. This is an example as stated by a new graduate many years ago, in 2004, to be precise.

"My very first code blue experience occurred 2 months into my hire here at this facility. It was a cold January morning and

I had just received report from the night shift RN and rounded on my assigned patients. One of them was an obese patient who was not doing so well until that morning, she sat bolt upright in bed and responded appropriately to my questions. A little while later, her doctor came around to see her and commented she was doing much better that morning, so I went on to see other patients. We had some student nurses for clinical experience on the floor that day and 2 were assigned to this patient. About half hour into the shift, the student nurses came running after me that my patient seemed to have stopped breathing, I rushed into her room to find that indeed she had stopped breathing, instead of dialing for code blue, I screamed for help, grabbed her ambu bag and started respiratory resuscitation. My colleagues heard me scream and dialed the code that had an instant response. Within minutes, the code blue team arrived and they took over the patient's resuscitation, sadly the patient died, but I remember I was shaken all day that being my very first code blue experience".

The above experience with different variations can be true for most new nurse graduates. Review of each code blue is done by an assigned team to learn what was done right and what not to do in subsequent cases- a learning experience for all.

It is worthwhile to stress the importance of teamwork in the clinical nursing practice. Where there is good teamwork the entire nursing team works together as one. When there is some slack, another team member can pick it up such that not one nursing staff is overwhelmed.

Teamwork fosters rapport among team members and may even prevent the burn-out syndrome that is often prevalent with nurses.

It is key for caregivers to constantly adhere to infection prevention practices as they perform their day-to-day activities. This will help achieve the desired outcomes set out in the plan of care and prevent common complications from hospitalization of patients.

CHAPTER FIVE

Infection Prevention

It is a well-known fact that hospitals are breeding grounds for cross infections or hospital acquired infections called nosocomial infections.

Evidence based practice promotes good hand hygiene to reduce the incidence to a large extent. For effective hand hygiene practice, there are five moments of hand hygiene that need to be observed by every caregiver as follows:

1. Before contact with patients:

   At this point, usually at the entrance to patient's room, there are hand hygiene products in the form of hand sanitizers or faucets to wash hands with.

   This ensures that the care giver is touching the patient with clean hands thus preventing possible contamination

2. Before embarking on clean/aseptic procedures: Again, because aseptic or sterile procedures must be done with clean hands before donning the sterile

gears, care givers must first wash their hands. The caregiver must also wash their hands at the end of the procedure.

3. After body fluid exposure:

   Body fluids include saliva, emesis, sweat, blood, fluids from open weepy wounds, tears, urine, semen, vaginal discharge, and bowel motions. Nurses and nursing assistants are the most exposed to patients' body fluids. Therefore, they must constantly wash their hands with soap and water after each exposure.

   However, hand hygiene is not limited to this group of caregivers. Everyone that meets patients is expected to commit to effective hand hygiene practice

4. After touching a patient:

   This is a continuum of hand hygiene practice in the care of patients, as they are the vulnerable group to protect. Regardless of how clean the patient may look, germs are not visible and the saying "prevention is better than cure" holds true. Special care must be taken to not overlook and skip hand washing at this point.

5. After touching patients' surroundings:

This is the last moment of good hand hygiene practice, as it is usually the last thing to do before leaving the patient's room.

It is when a nurse tidies up the room, makes the bed, or makes the patient comfortable in bed by repositioning. The caregiver touches the patient's surroundings almost every time one enters a patient's room. Whatever the chore is, hands must be washed or cleansed with hand sanitizer before leaving the room. This allows one to enter the next patient with clean hands and also prevent contaminating one another, (http://www.who.int > cleanhands)

The above is standard precaution for infection prevention in caring for all patients. Some patients will need other forms of precautions taken for their specific condition as indicated by their diagnosis.

Lessons from Florence Nightingale.

Florence Nightingale is known as the pioneer of modern nursing practice as demonstrated by her care of wounded soldiers in the Crimean war. She found correlation between the patients who died and their environmental conditions conditions (www.nursing-theory.org > nightingale). This informed the environmental theory in modern nursing practice. Her nurses cleaned the whole hospital so there was limited amount of germs helping to stop contamination and spread of disease. (https://myhero.com > f¬¬_Nightingale) .

No wonder evidence-based practice today recommends that hand washing in addition to the clean environment in hospitals will result in similar outcomes.

In line with Nightingale's environment of care is her passion for caring for sick soldiers. It takes a measure of devotion and love for the RN to care for all categories of patients. As in the healthy individual with varying human character, the sick also exhibit different characteristics and responses to sickness. There is what is commonly referred to as the "difficult patient" by nurses, where regardless of all care given, the patient remained unsatisfied or unhappy. Oftentimes, there may be underlying psychological factors that drive this behavior and need to be identified and dealt with for the patient to cooperate with care.

Here is an example of "difficult" patient. Due to risk for infection, retention of a Foley catheter for longer than 72hrs from insertion is discouraged except when contraindicated.

A patient was admitted from another facility with an indwelling catheter with no indication to continue, and the receiving nurse proceeded to discontinue it as was the protocol in her facility. The patient absolutely refused to have it taken out and the nurse left her alone citing patient's right.

Several other nurses also tried on their shifts with the same result.

A compassionate nurse who sat with the patient, talked with the patient and found out why she did not want the catheter removed. The nurse discovered that the patient was afraid that she would wet herself from accidental incontinence without the Foley. This nurse developed a plan to come in to take her to the bathroom every hour to prevent that accident. The patient agreed to the care. The Foley was taken out and the nurse took care of the bathroom visits throughout the shift.

The patient was happy and gave excellent remarks about the nurse- a win –win situation.

This example illustrates the need for the RN to go the extra mile to provide the best care.

In addition to clinical practice, the RN is expected to be involved in extracurricular activities one of which is volunteering

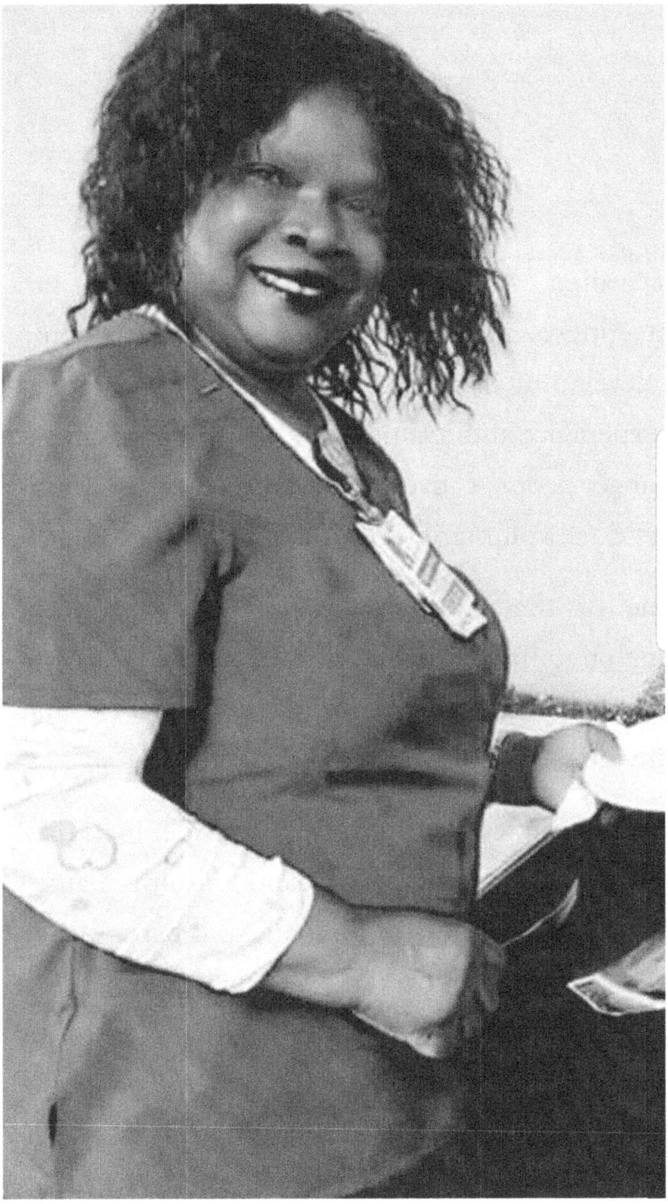

CHAPTER SIX

Volunteering

According to excerpts from megaessays.com, volunteering is a way of giving back to your community while developing important social skills and gaining valuable work experience at the same time. It gives one an opportunity to change people's lives including your own. They are services done voluntarily without expecting a pay

One of the expectations of a RN is volunteering. Although not mandatory, many areas of need exist where the RN can volunteer hours, expertise, or money. It could be on an individual basis or corporately.

Some examples of volunteering include: food drives, the various Health Foundations, and Health Fairs. Some churches have Health Fairs annually and participation. One could also sign up for races in support of the various Foundations. Another area of participation is Jury duty. This is mandatory for every citizen that is so summoned, and where the date clashes with work, the individual is given priority to attend over work.

Many committees exist in the workplace and all Registered Nurses are expected to belong to at least one and be actively involved in their¬¬ activities. This has a positive reflection on the person's yearly evaluation and could be one of the criteria looked at for pay raise during evaluations.

Corporately, some facilities adopt a foundation to participate in on a yearly basis and expect all members of staff to contribute time or money. To adopt a foundation, forums exist for staff members to come together to make decisions on which one is preferred. When a decision is made, usually by majority, the foundation becomes the choice for that year and work begins through to the next year. It involves participation from all departments of the facility and is one of the interdisciplinary networks that exists in some health care facilities.

CHAPTER SEVEN

Interdisciplinary Relationship

Nursing and nurses do not exist in isolation. Although they are usually the largest workforce at any healthcare facility, they work with other healthcare departments within the facility.

Nurses are in patients' environment 24/7. They interact with doctors, laboratory staff, radiology staff, dietary staff, engineering (maintenance) staff, house- keeping staff, security staff, family, transportation and even with staff from other facilities, on behalf of the patient.

Nurses coordinate the care of patients with multiple disciplines/departments and ensure that nothing is missed or overlooked. They become teachers to patients as they explain the different procedures ordered for them from the different disciplines and the expected outcomes.

Nurses receive patients from transporters when they come and go from other departments for procedures or when they are freshly admitted to the floor. In fulfilling these roles, the RN has the opportunity to get to know the patients and develop rapport with them and their families. Patients also come to trust the nurse and depend on him/her for care.

The World Health organization (WHO) describes health as the state of complete physical, mental, and social well-being and not merely the absence of disease or infirmity, and the fundamental right of every human being (WHO, 1946). For this reason, a patient in the hospital needs total holistic care of the physical, mental and social state. This involves a multidisciplinary approach from the various healthcare departments with the RN coordinating these activities of care.

Imagine a situation where a patient is unable to care for himself, he will need total nursing care, he is not alert, cannot speak, move, eat or drink for himself, yet needs all these human functions met.

The RN is responsible to feed the patient through an appropriate mode of feeding determined by the doctor and/or recommended by the nutritionist.

The RN ensures that the patient does not develop pressure sores that so commonly happen when one stays in the same position for too long and circulation is cut off from the area. The RN frequently turns and reassesses the body parts during turning to make sure the skin is still intact.

The nurse also ensures that that patient is not dirty from urine or bowel motion as the patient is incontinent and cannot control his bladder or bowel. The RN must clean the patient and if necessary may have to do a bed bath. Having done all these, there is still one vital care missing- mouth care.

In a healthy patient, not daily brushing the teeth gives off a bad odor called halitosis, imagine then the odor in an unresponsive patient that does not have mouth care done frequently. This care is often missed in such patients and calls for more attention and diligence. It is part of the care of patients that are totally dependent for care.

Because the RN stays with patients longer than any other member of the care team, he/she is better placed to note the changing conditions of the patient for the better or worse. The nurse can therefore advocate for the needs of the patient and effect their implementation, for positive outcomes.

CHAPTER EIGHT

The Nurse as an Advocate.

Of the many responsibilities of the RN is that of Advocacy. Wikipedia describes advocacy as the activity of an individual or group which aims to influence decisions within political, economic, and social systems and institutions. The realm of influence of the RN therefore falls within social, economic, and health systems and institutions.

Sometimes patients come in from the streets, that is they are homeless, the RN refers such patients to the social worker. The social worker will work with the patient on finding a place for them on discharge as well as arranging transportation and even clothing to ensure that the patient's basic needs are met.

While on admission, the RN uses her judgement to identify patient's areas of need during assessments. The nurse help to meet the patients' needs and ensures consultation with physicians or other appropriate healthcare team members for such needs to be met.

During communication with physicians, the nurse recommends the best line of action to care for the patient according to his/her assessment of the patient's current situation. And keeping in mind what would best serve the patient.

The RN puts him/herself in the place of the patients and treats them as he/she would have his/her family member treated in difficult situations of hospitalization.

A simple example includes a RN seeing a patient having difficulty feeding. The RN needs to determine what is causing the difficulty; is the patient unable to chew because portions are too big, or does the patient not have his/ her dentures or is the patient too weak to eat? The RN determines the cause and takes actions to remedy it. The remedy may include informing the physician that the patient needs a nutrition consultation. The nurse will then follow through to see that the problem is resolved. Subsequent meals should be appropriate for patient such that he/she is able to feed self freely or assisted to feed without any apparent or perceived risk.

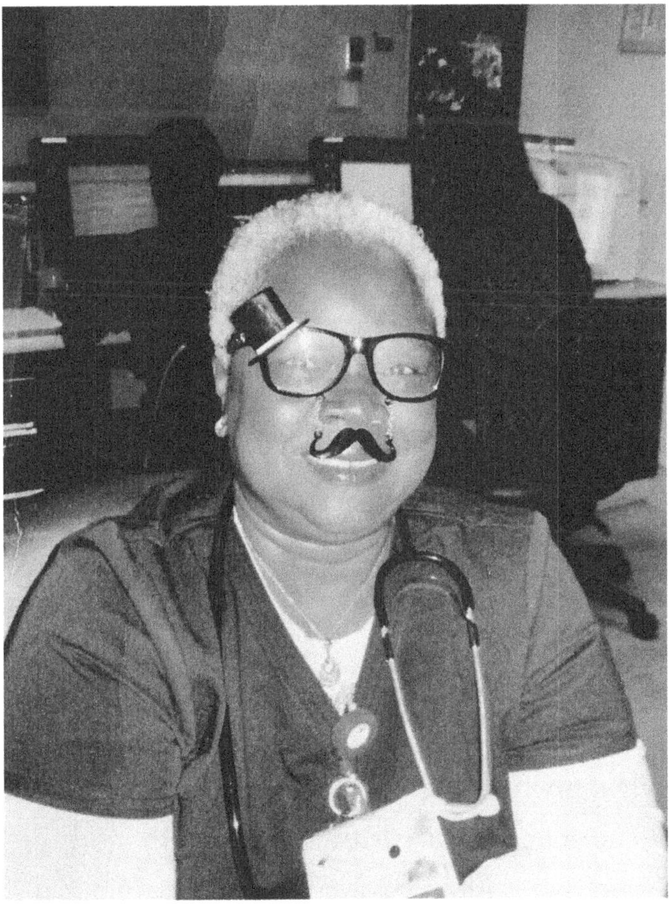

CHAPTER NINE

Work-Life Balance

The saying that "all work and no play ......" holds true today and the place of recreation and rest from work cannot be overemphasized. This is an important aspect of policy in most healthcare facilities that drives the practice to self-schedule.

Team members fill in days/nights they want to work, and the charge nurse ensures that the unit is well covered while accommodating staff requests and schedules. Some facilities encourage staff members to live healthy lifestyles by providing exercise options, encourage smoking cessation and promote weight loss. Some facilities even provide massages in the workplace for their staff.

Each individual also has different prevailing situations and circumstances that need balancing with work. It is for this reason that staff are allowed to self-schedule that results in ease to comply, good staff retention ratio, and reduction in incidence of truancy.

In addition to teamwork, the other aspect that makes for work enjoyment is proper work-life balance. Records show many staff members that worked for up to 45years in any one facility, testified that work colleagues have become like family, and that kept them working in the same place. At some point though, there comes the need to retire, then what next?

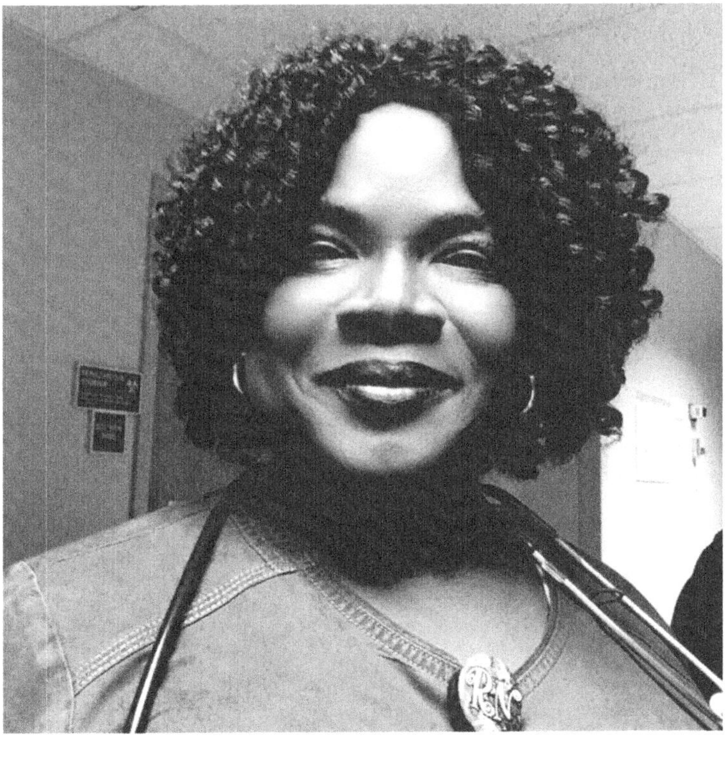

CHAPTER TEN

What Next

Do nurses ever retire you may ask?

Those that do not have any disabilities or physical impairments over the years have increasingly had difficulty quitting nursing practice completely. The average retirement age for nurses is the late 60s according to "nurse Michelle, Dec 2003".

The insurance factor makes it difficult for nurses in this category to retire. Most nurses find that retirement will rob them of health insurance coverage. It is at this time of life that most people have health challenges, and to not have health insurance could be suicidal.

Leaving clinical practice or bedside nursing as it is more commonly known, for less physically demanding areas of practice is therefore the next option for this category of nurses.

Some nurses may find it more convenient at this point in their career to mentor or encourage the younger generation of nurses. By sharing their own experiences of nursing with the up and coming nurses is a way to pay it forward.

CHAPTER ELEVEN

Pay It Forward

At this time of life, nurses have finished raising their families (children, for those that have families) and have become grandparents. They now have the unique function of influencing the career path of people in their circle of influence, unwittingly, paying forward the profession within their family or community.

It is not uncommon to find generations of nurses within a family from great grandparent to grandparent to parent and down the line, in circles entirely outside of family, in areas like the church or other close-knit communities. This can also be true for other professions and may not necessarily be the sequence to pay it forward, however the saying that "once a nurse, always a nurse" holds true for most nurses whether active or retired. Often nurses find themselves in activities directly or remotely connected to nursing.

Nursing is a noble profession and kudos to all nurses.

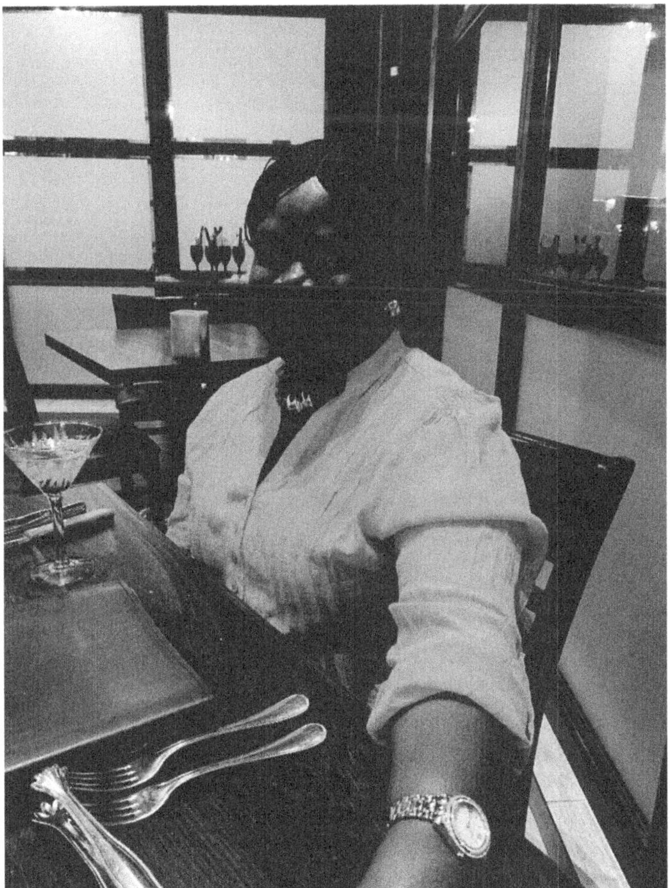

BIBLIOGRAPHY

1. NurseJournal.org, 2019
2. WHO, 1946
3. http://www.who.int > cleanhands
4. www.nursing-theory.org > nightingale
5. https://myhero.com > f_Nightingale
6. nursemichelle, 2003.

ABOUT THE AUTHOR

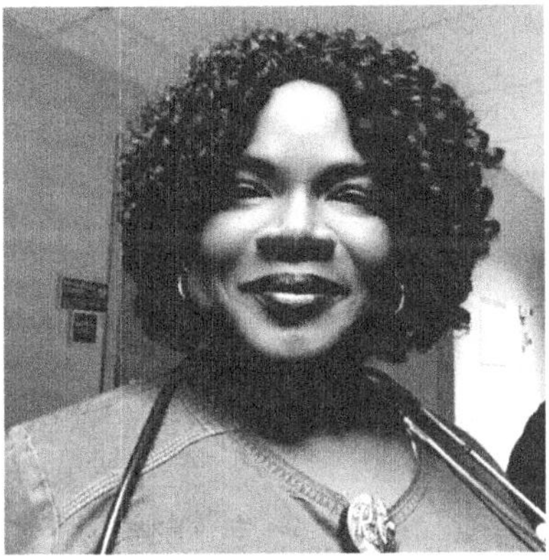

Anne Dada is an accomplished leader in the Nursing field. She is a Registered Nurse with over 40years' experience in Clinical Nursing Practice. She has worked in different departments; Medical-Surgical, Neuro-Trauma and the Special care units. She is a Naturalized American, originally from Nigeria in Africa. She is also a born-again Christian, joyfully serving the Lord in her community and her local church. She lives happily with her husband, Kola and they are blessed with four beautiful children-Oluwagbotemi, Oluwadamilare, Oluwabukunmi, and Oluwadamilola and grandchildren.

REVIEWS

Nursing is a compassionate profession. Your heart must be in it to write this beautiful piece for not only the newly registered, but also for those that are willing to learn more. My friend and auntie has put in writing her wealth of experience as a nurse in this booklet. I recommend it to all.

Earnest Okonofua, RN

THOUGHTS

Made in the USA
Monee, IL
08 November 2026

68002502R00038